AYURVEDA

The science of Life!

Cover & Graphic Design

Mattias Långström

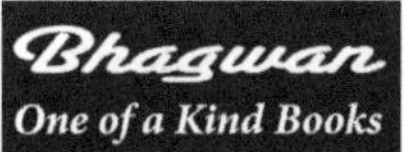

AYURVEDA

The science of Life!

ISBN 9789198735819

✺✺✺

Copyright © Mattias Långström

Publisher: **BHAGWAN 2022**

No part of this publication may be reproduced or transmitted in any form, or by any means, electronic or mechanical, including photocopying, scanning, recording, or any information storage and retrieval sýstem, without express written permission from the publisher, except for the inclusion of brief quotations embodied in critical articles and reviews. This book is a work of fiction and a product of the author´s imagination.

Namasté

I want to thank the teachers and students I have had over the years and who have made my journey with yoga so interesting. Thank you for all the inspiration you have given me and for making this book possible. The yoga masters who no longer live among us, live on with every new person who immerses themselves in the yoga tradition.

Sri Swami Sivananda, Sri Swami Satyananda, Sri Tiru-malai Krishnamacharya, Sri Swami Vishnudevananda, Sri K. Pattabhi Jois, Osho, Swami Nirdosha, Swami Omananda, Swami Janakananda, Ole Schmidt, Turiya, Maryam Abrishami and Sanna Kuittinen.

Everyone who has searched for answers to what they perceived through an activated ajna chakra. In yoga, they have learned the principles behind the universe, the collective consciousness, and the creative power, Kunda-lini Shakti. The duality behind everything, both what we see and what we do not see. Together we help to pass on the previous secret knowledge, about our gunas, nadis, and chakras, to anyone who wants to be seen.

THE AUTHOR

Shreyananda Natha is the author of over twelve titles on yoga. Among other things, he has written the most comprehensive books on yoga in Swedish – Everything About Yoga and the study book The Yoga Bible. He is also a certified yoga and meditation teacher according to EYTF's international guidelines and has undergone a multi-year yoga teacher training under the leadership of Swami Omananda at Satyananda Ashram. Shreyananda Natha holds the highest initiation in the Tantric Natha Order. He travels frequently to Asia and India to improve himself, and to gain knowledge and inspiration. He has immersed himself in the tantric rituals and is known for his extensive knowledge of yoga, deep relaxation, and meditation

There is no authority that can say what yoga is. When you give yourself fully and completely, and experience yoga without limitations or doubts, when you become one with the true experience in yourself, the real encounter with yoga arises. Only then do you understand what yoga is – for you. You are no longer limited by ornament, shyness and artificial thought patterns that lie as a filter between you and the transformation. Yoga is a cultural-historical wealth that is still passed on from teacher to student and helps man to find his way back to his true nature. It opens us up and attracts awareness.

It strengthens our self-esteem, and our entire person's spectrum of possibilities suddenly becomes visible to us. Yoga is not difficult. You do not have to be vegan or able to stand on your head. You just need to practice your yoga regularly and the rest will come by itself.

With all the love from the universe – Aum Shanti Shreyananda Natha.

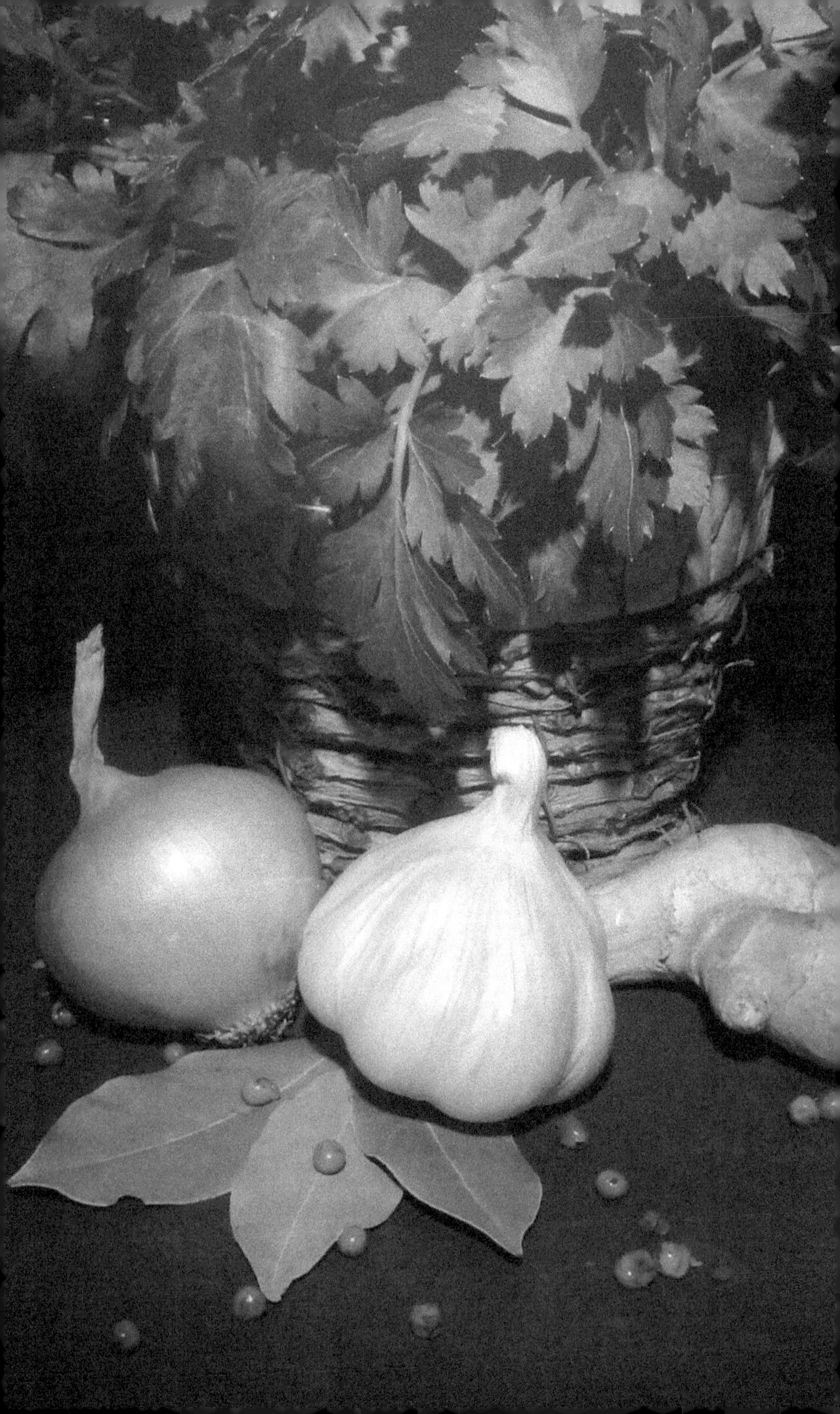

AYURVEDA

VATA, PITTA & KAPHA

Ayurveda is an Indian health science with roots in the Vedic tradition. Both yoga and Ayurveda originally came into being as Vedic teachings and are believed to be more than five thousand years old.

Ayur means life and Veda means knowledge – the knowledge/science about life. With the help of Ayurveda, we can learn to live in balance with our life force and our entire divine consciousness.

In Ayurveda, the whole person is treated, not just the sick. When you create balance, you simultaneously release the self-healing forces. Ayurveda develops the health potential we have within us and at the same time expands our consciousness.

Ayurveda and yoga originate from the same tradition and have been practiced together for thousands of years. This is often forgotten resulting in yoga and Ayurveda being taught separately. Both classical yoga and Ayurveda take the whole person into account, physically, mentally and spiritually.

You could say that Ayurveda is a tradition of Vedic

knowledge that describes how to heal the body and mind while yoga is a tradition of Vedic knowledge that describes the path to self-insight. Achieving self-insight requires that the body and mind are in balance.

UPAVEDAS

Ayurveda is part of the four upavedas that supplement the four Vedas. Ayurveda is also closely related to the practice of Veda as it treats various mantras and methods to cure diseases.

The four upavedas are:

1. Ayurveda – knowledge of life.

2. Gandharva veda – knowledge of the role of culture, art and music for spiritual development. For example, there is music for various disease conditions.

3. Dhanur veda – knowledge of the importance of behavior for spiritual development.

4. Sthapatya veda – knowledge of the importance of architecture for spiritual development. This veda is also known as vastu and is reminiscent of feng shui. Feng Shui is a philosophy which practices arranging building structures and objects within living spaces to create balance and energy.

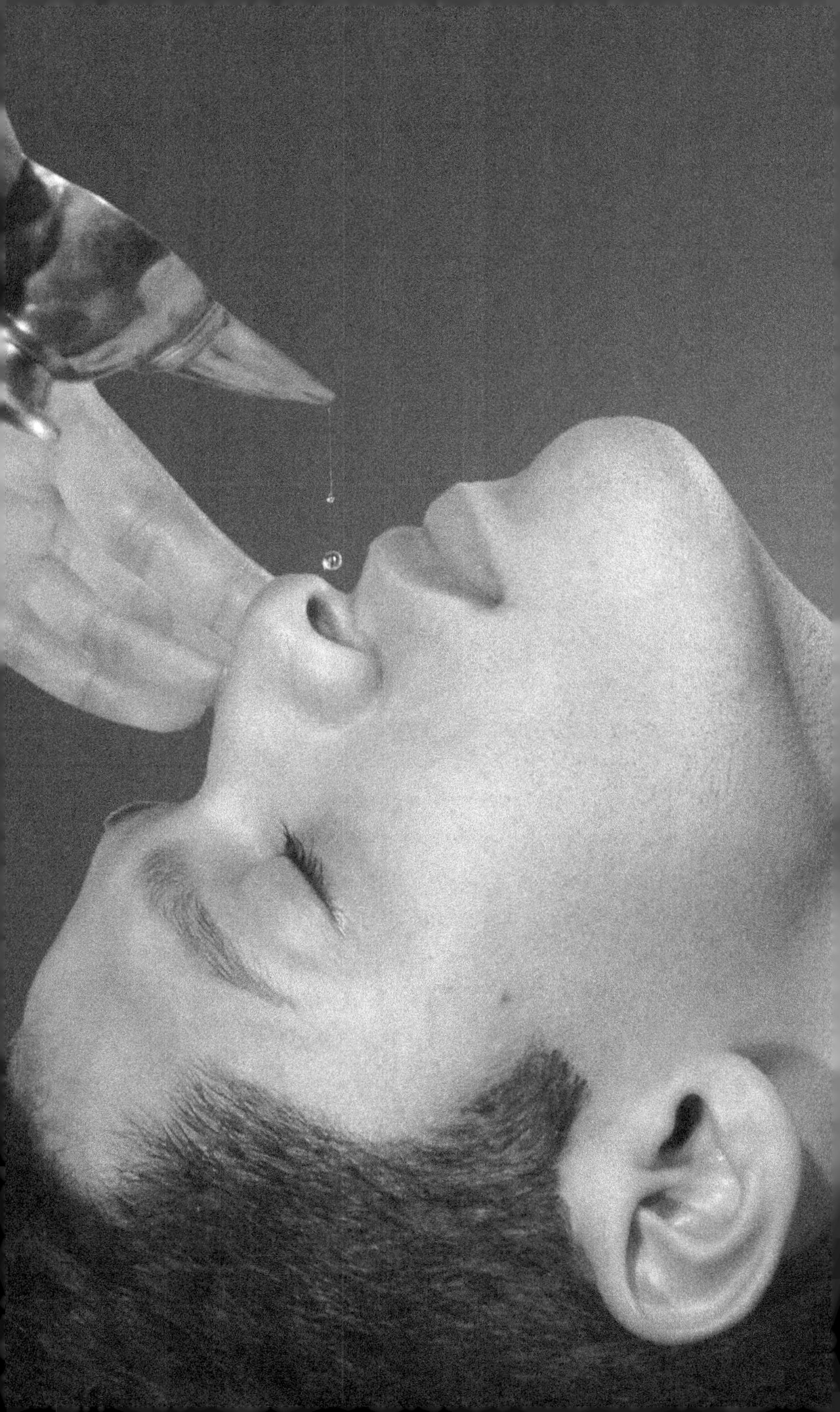

THREE DOSHAS

In Ayurveda, there are three doshas or energy principles which control all life processes both internally and externally. Our entire biological existence is based on the interplay between these three energy principles. Doshas are a combination of the five elements: space, air, fire, water and earth.

The doshas also determine what personality type you are. It is usually said that you have one or two doshas that dominate. According to astrology, it is the influence of the celestial bodies (grahas) during the conception that determines which dosha becomes the most dominant in each person. There is dosha type one, dosha type two and dosha type three.

In our yoga practice, it is important to understand how the doshas affect us. When we understand the energy principles and how they affect and interact in and around us, we can take full advantage of the fine yogic techniques to create balance and harmony in our physical and subtle body. We can adapt our yoga practice to the needs and personality type that we are to achieve the best possible results.

In Ayurveda, yoga is used as a basis for maintaining a healthy lifestyle but also as a treatment method for dis-

*eases. Asanas, pranayamas and meditation are among
the best methods to maintain balance in the doshas.*

VATA	**PITTA**	**KAPHA**
Space/air.	*Fire/water.*	*Water/soil.*
Movement.	*Combustion.*	*Structure.*
Dry.	*A little oily.*	*Fat/oily.*
Light.	*Light.*	*Heavy.*
Cold.	*Warm/hot.*	*Cold.*
Very fast.	*Fast.*	*Slow.*
Hearing/feeling.	*The eyes.*	*Taste/smell.*
The moon.	*The sun.*	*Earth.*

*Vata is kinetic energy in all kinds of ways and the force
that allows the other two doshas to move. Vata exists as
air in our organs, joints and bones. On a deeper level,
vata is the life force within us and the power of thought
that moves in our mind. Vata controls the central nervous system, the movements of the heart, the intestines,*

the lungs, the thought processes and the communication between the mind and the body.

Pitta is responsible for the metabolism and conversion process in the body. In addition to digestion, it also melts our impressions from the outside world, emotions and ideas. Pitta provides us with intelligence, courage and vitality. Without pitta, we lose motivation and sight to reach our goals in life. In nature, you can see pitta in photosynthesis, which is nature's combustion.

Kapha is the one who unites. . It is the stable structure that is associated with bone structure, mucous membranes and joints in the body and rocks and mountains in nature. Kapha provides us with emotions and feelings that contribute to love, care, devotion and faith which causes us to both maintain harmony within ourselves and to unite with others.

Vata, pitta and *kapha* are closely linked and always work together. In every single cell in the body, these three interact. In order for vata to be in balance, it is necessary that pitta and kapha exist in the right proportion because it has these two elements in it in the form of water and fire. Vata is easiest to get out of balance, but it is also the easiest to rebalance. Pitta in turn needs to be watered with vata's properties of movement and *decomposition (start the fire/dampen the fire) and also kapha's building and preserving properties to keep the fire alive. Kapha needs vata to start the movement and pitta for its stimulus and warming properties. Consequently, we see that none of the doshas can exist without the other; they are all equally important.*

RAJAS, TAMAS & SATTVA

Prakriti consists of three varying qualities: rajas, tamas and sattva. Rajas is the active, stimulating and positive force that contributes to change. Tamas is the passive and negative force that keeps the old. Sattva is the neutral and balancing force that harmonizes the positive and the negative. All three energies are necessary in everything that happens, even on the spiritual plane.

Sattva is the light, the love and the life. It is the higher spiritual power that makes us develop our consciousness. Rajas is the passion, the twilight and what changes. It is the vital force that lacks stability. It gives rise to emotional fluctuations such as fear and desire, love and hate. Tamas is the dark, the insensitive, and the dead. It is the lower material force that pulls us down to unconsciousness, stagnation, listlessness and heaviness. Unmanifested Prakriti keeps these three in balance. Rajas and tamas get sattva together. When Prakriti is manifested, these qualities are distinguished.

Sattva gives rise to the mind, rajas generates the life force and tamas stands for form and substance as the physical body. Yoga and Ayurveda want to develop the sattvic state. In yoga, sattva is the higher quality that makes us develop spiritually. In Ayurveda, sattva is the state of balance in which the healing property is released.

YOGIC AND AYURVEDIC DIET

In Ayurveda, diet plays a very big role and lays the foundation for all other therapeutic approaches and healing processes. Without a proper and balanced diet, other medicines have no major effect. The food is used as medicine. A sattvic diet is advocated because sattva creates balance. A sattvic diet is traditionally based on ahimsa, which is an ethical principle of not causing harm to other living beings. The food should, as far as possible, have been allowed to grow naturally in a harmonious environment as such food carries a lot of prana and pure awareness.

Yogis around the world are usually very aware of what they are eating but a traditional yogic diet and an Ayurvedic one are different. Ayurveda wants to create balance and build good physical health. In yoga, you want to develop and change body awareness. In short: Ayurveda wants to create physical health and yoga helps us to get beyond the limits of the body. Many traditional yogic paths are ascetic in nature where solid, simple raw foods with detoxifying effects are common. However, these have a water-raising effect. Traditional Ayurvedic diet is instead based on a well-cooked and nutritious food in order to strengthen us physically and prevent any of the doshas from becoming unbalanced and or unnecessarily wet.

A traditional yogic diet increases the elements of space/ ether and air(vata) in order to detoxify and open up the mind. Therefore, raw food and fasting are recommended. By reducing the body, you expand the mind. Another significant factor in the yogic diet is prana. A raw diet is rich in prana. By following a raw diet, you increase the flow of prana in the body and thus purify nadis. Breathing exercises are used to increase the digestive fire in the body, which allows the food to be digested even though it's not cooked.

However, few of us are able to digest this type of food satisfactorily. This is especially true for vata people who have a varying digestive fire, but even kapha and pitta can have difficulty with this. Therefore, most non-ascetics feel better from a well-cooked, warm diet that is easy to digest.

An Ayurvedic diet is not necessarily sattvic, but is more focussed on creating physical health. A Yogic diet, on the other hand, places the greatest emphasis on the food's satiety, which can increase a dosha. For an optimal diet, you can choose sattvic food that is adapted to your dominant dosha type. Sattvic food includes: dairy products, natural oils, herbal teas, sweet spices, fruits, fresh juices, vegetables, cereals, legumes, nuts, seeds and honey. For a sattvic diet, it is important to eat the right type of food at the right time during the day because the day is also divided into vata, pitta and kapha time. In Ayurveda, it is recommended to eat light food for breakfast because Kapha time prevails and heavy food weighs down the mind and body as well. The biggest goal should be to eat in the middle of the day during pitta time when digestion is at its strongest. In the evening, you should not eat heavy foods or t too close to bedtime as it disturbs both sleep and the natural cleansing of waste materials.

THE SIX TASTES
There are six different flavors that affect each dosha in different ways. Each flavor consists of a combination of two elements.

Sweet – water and soil.
Balances vata and pitta. Increases kapha. For example, vegetables, oils, milk and rice.

Sour – fire and soil.
Balances vata. Increases pitta and kapha. For example,
citrus, yogurt, cheese and vinegar.

Salt – fire and water.
Balances vata. Increases pitta and kapha. For example,
seaweed, tamari, table salt.

Pungent – fire and air.
Decreases kapha. Increases pitta and vata. For example,
strong spices such as pepper, onion and ginger.

Bitter – space and air.
Balances pitta and kapha. Increases vata. For example,
green leafy vegetables and turmeric.

Astringent – air and soil.
Balances pitta and kapha. Increases vata. For example,
beans, lentils and unripe bananas.

TIP
Try to eat in silence and in a relaxed manner. Focus
on the meal and not on anything else at the same time.
Eat foods you like and avoid cold foods. Avoid eating
when you feel anxious, angry or sad. Drink boiled water
with food, not milk. Eat freshly prepared food as much
as possible and avoid leftovers, as the nutrients have
already been lost. The food must be prepared with love
and awareness.

AGNI

In Ayurveda, the body's digestive fire – called agni, is of great importance. If the fire is too weak, the food cannot be digested satisfactorily and nutrients are lost. The food we eat then instead turns into ama(slag products) which strains our body. In Ayurveda, a weak digestive fire is seen as the root cause of most diseases. Our modern life and the stress we live with are major contributing factors to poor digestion. We tend to gulp down food instead of enjoying it.

When we have balance between the doshas, the agni will also be in balance. A sign of this is when we feel a healthy appetite at regular times.

The agni is weakened when we overeat, snack or eat even though we are not hungry. Refrigerated food, long fasting and poorly chewed food are also contributing factors.

When vata is increased, digestion becomes irregular. It can change from fast to slow and sometimes you can feel a strong hunger and sometimes nothing at all. Stomach problems are also part of the picture.

When pitta gets out of balance, the agni becomes too strong. You may experience a very strong hunger, often shortly after eating. This contributes to nutrients not being absorbed by the body and in the long run you can suffer from stomach ulcers.

When kapha is elevated, digestion becomes very slow instead. You experience a heavy feeling after eating and feelings of hunger are weak.

AGNI YOGA

Both yoga and Ayurveda carry the knowledge of the divine fire, the agni. We learn to control the fire in order to create balance and to develop. The cosmic fire exists everywhere; in ourselves and around us. In the body, we see the agni in the form of our digestive fire, and on a finer level, the agni corresponds to our eternal consciousness. Without fire, our development and evolution will stop.

In Ayurveda, we learn to balance the function of the agni physically by taking care of our digestive fire, which then lays the foundation for good health.

In yoga the focus is on the pranic agni and the fire of meditation, both of which are important for our path to enlightenment. Various fire rituals are common in yoga traditions, but we may be most familiar with the Breath of Fire exercise, which cleanses the body's energy channels and increases the flow of prana in the body.

YOGAS IMPACT ON OUR THREE DOSHAS

ASANAS AND AYURVEDA

Asanas release tension and energy blockages that may have occurred, thereby keeping the body's tissues, joints and organs in the best possible shape. The positions stretch and strengthen the muscles, and the spine is kept flexible, making it possible for the energy to flow freely through nerves that belong to our organs and glands. Our tissues are therefore cleansed in a systematic way, which prepares the body for the more advanced yogic exercises.

Asanas prepare you for breathing exercises and meditation. They not only have a physical purpose but they also affect us on a practical, mental and spiritual level. Asanas have from the beginning aimed to counter rajas, the turbulent energy within us that distracts the mind.

Asanas help to balance and release the prana in the body, which prepares us for the breathing exercises. Our senses are turned inward which facilitates mind control (pratyahara). When our thoughts are still, the mind is calmed so that we can concentrate (dharana) and meditate (dhyana).

Diet and asanas are the two most important factors in creating good health and, in the long run, counteracting imbalances and diseases.

To balance the prana in the body, spices, herbs and various breathing exercises are used. To enable this, a proper posture and diet are required as a basis. Our posture is of great importance for our health and consciousness. The body and the mind influence each other through subtle channels in the body through which foods and our thoughts flow. The channels are held together by the musculoskeletal system, the shape of which is determined by our posture. Improper posture causes stress in the body and blocks these channels. The energy cannot flow optimally and residual products and toxins get a chance to accumulate. This eventually leads to discomfort in the body, pain and illness.

It is easy for asanas to become the mainstay of yoga practice. If you want to take part in yoga on a deeper level, you should give equal time to asanas, pranayamas and meditation. An exaggerated and unconscious execution of asanas leads to a fixation on the body and boosts our physical ego: this leads to a rigid and undeveloped mind and emotions. Never exaggerate the exercises or force the body into a position, which will only cause more tension and injury.

ASANAS AND OUR AGE

Infants and children are by nature soft and flexible in the body. Starting to practice asanas at an early age means that you maintain the softness and correct posture for life.

At the age of sixty-five – which is the vata age, the body fluids slowly begin to decrease and dry out. The body becomes stiffer and joint diseases are common. With the help of asanas, you can keep your body in shape and balance excess vata.

Vinyasas are suitable for younger people because a lot of rajas prevail in body and mind and they need vinyasas to mature. After the age of twenty-four, one should move on to inner yoga and develop the mind by studying yogic texts.

After the age of forty-eight, the mind develops at the same speed as the physical energies are withdrawn. You should spend more time meditating but asanas are still important for keeping the body supple and healthy.

At the age of seventy-two, the mind develops even more. This is the time for deep meditation. Asanas continue to be important to slow down aging.

ASANAS FOR VATA

Vata people often have a slim and thin physique. They are very flexible and mobile when young but easily develop stiffness as they age. Vatas often suffer from joint problems at middle age. They are often cold, have dry skin, cracked joints, and poor blood circulation. Vata people are naturally nervous and scared, which makes them tense in their shoulders and back. Asanas are very important for vata people, for both their health and their ability to meditate. Vatas must exercise caution when practicing asanas as they are prone to injury. Soft, flowing exercises at a reasonable speed are preferred.

Mental preparation is important for vatas: a moment of rest and deep breathing before asanas is a must. During the actual practice, vatas should start slowly so the circulation awakens and the joints have a chance to warm up. Vatas should not be too sweaty as they dry out easily. Intake of fluid is important. Asanas should mainly affect the area around the hips and intestines which is the main seat of vata. Releasing tension from the hips and lumbar spine is important. Too much stretching and movement can cause over-stretching and weakness.

Sitting positions are good for vata such as padmasana and vajrasana. These have a calming, grounding effect and control apana vayu.

Keeping the spine flexible is important for vatas who often accumulate tension here. Exercises that rotate the spine in each direction are good. Matsyendrasana is an example of a pose which releases vata from the nervous system. It is important to have proper breathing when performing spinal rotation, otherwise the pose will have the opposite effect and increase vata.

Forward bending positions have a calming effect and release vata from the back. Combining forward bending positions with backward bending positions is important to maximize the benefits. However, this should be done slowly and carefully. Doing backward bending positions too quickly can stimulate the sympathetic nervous system and our "fight or flight" mechanism. With caution, asanas such as the cobra and the grasshopper have a grounding and strengthening effect on vatas.

Standing poses are very good for vata. They build strength, give peace and increase stability.

Vatas should avoid becoming too exhausted. Dynamic asanas should be accompanied by sitting positions in combination with pranayamas and meditation.

After asanas, vatas should lie and rest in shavasana. It is an optimal time to meditate, with the mind calm and the emotions stable.

Seated poses:
Siddhasana/siddha yoni asana(perfect pose), vajrasana (diamond pose) and simhasana (lion pose).

The sun salutation:
Slowly and consciously.

Standing poses:
Vrksasana (tree pose), trikonasana (triangle pose), virabhadrasana (warrior pose), parighasana (gate pose) and all standing forward bending positions.

Inverted poses:
Shirshasana (headstand), vipareeta karani asana (half shoulder stand).

Backbends:
Bhujangasana (cobra) and shalabhasana (grasshopper).

Forward bends:
All. Especially janu sirsasana (half butterfly) and pachimottasana (pliers).

Spinal twists:
Lying positions, bharadvajasana (half turn) and shava udarakarshanasana (universal position).

Other:
Shashankasana (hare), parivrtta janu sirsasana
(one-legged forward bend in a seated position), navasa-
na (boat), yoga mudra.

Shavasana:
At least twenty minutes.

ASANAS FOR PITTA

Pittas have a medium-sized physique. They often have good muscles and flexibility. Circulation and joint mobility are usually good due to the slightly oily nature of pittas. Pittas usually handle asanas very well, but if overdone, it may lead to hypermobility and stiffness in joints.

Mentally, pitta people are aggressive and like to shine in everything they do. Pittas must be careful about "performing" when it comes to asanas. They can often become very good at the technical part but forget about the spiritual part. Pittas are often overambitious, annoyed and very driven. Asanas should be used to cool pittas down both physically and mentally, thereby helping them turn the intelligence inward to better understand themselves.

Calm breathing and sitting still after powerful asanas are important to counteract any stress. Pittas should avoid overly strenuous exercise and not get too hot. Powerful asanas are ok as long as pittas compensate by using cooling asanas and pranayamas to cool the mind and body towards the end.

Around the navel, heat is created and distributed throughout the body. In the palate where saliva is secreted, we have a cooling function in the body. The heat from the umbilical region moves upwards in order to reduce the cold produced in the soft palate. By standing in a shoulder position or entering the plow position, the cooling property is protected from the heat. These positions reverse the positions of the sun and the moon in the body, which creates balance especially in pitta people. Spinal twists such as matsyendrasana are also good for protecting the cooling property without lowering the fire in the body. Positions that release tension and affect the abdominal tract, small intestine and liver are also beneficial for pittas because pitta accumulates in these areas. The bow, cobra, boat and fish poses are good. Headstand increases pitta and should be avoided if you do not know how to balance the heat afterwards.

Forward bending positions are generally good for pittas because they increase the energy around the abdomen, have a cooling effect and also a grounding effect.

Back-bending positions create more heat and should therefore be practiced in moderation and followed by cooling asanas. Seated spinal twists help cleanse the liver and detoxify the pitta.

After asanas, pitta should feel calm, cool and relaxed in the stomach. The mind should be in a meditative state and not too sharp.

Seated poses:
Most are beneficial except simhasana(the lion) which should be avoided.

The moon greeting:
Cooling for pitta.

Standing poses:
Vrksasana(tree pose), trikonasana(triangle pose), ardha chandrasana(crescent pose).

Standing poses(legs wide apart):
Moordhasana(head on the floor from standing with legs apart), padottanasana(leg lift).

Forward bends:
All seated forward bends are good, especially pada pra-sar paschimottanasana(forward bend with legs split), kurmasana(turtle) and paschimottanasana(pliers).

Twists:
Ardha matsyendrasana(half spinal rotation).

Other:
Sarvangasana(shoulder stand), vipareeta karani(half shoulder stand), navasana(boat), ardha matsyendrasana(seated spine twisting), bhujangasana(cobra), yoga mudra.

Shavasana:
Medium, long.

ASANAS FOR KAPHA

Kapha types are heavily built and gain weight easily. They are often inflexible and should not try to push the body into a position like the lotus position, which carries a risk of injury. Kapha's body and joints often do not support these positions. Kaphas must accept how they are built and not try to become thin slim yogis, because their body is not built that way.

Kapha women can be thin when they are young but gain weight over the years, especially after giving birth. This can weigh down kaphas as they may have a hard time accepting this. It is then common in this case for them to use different ways to try to lose weight such as yoga although it rarely gives results. Kaphas must instead work on their attitude toward their body and

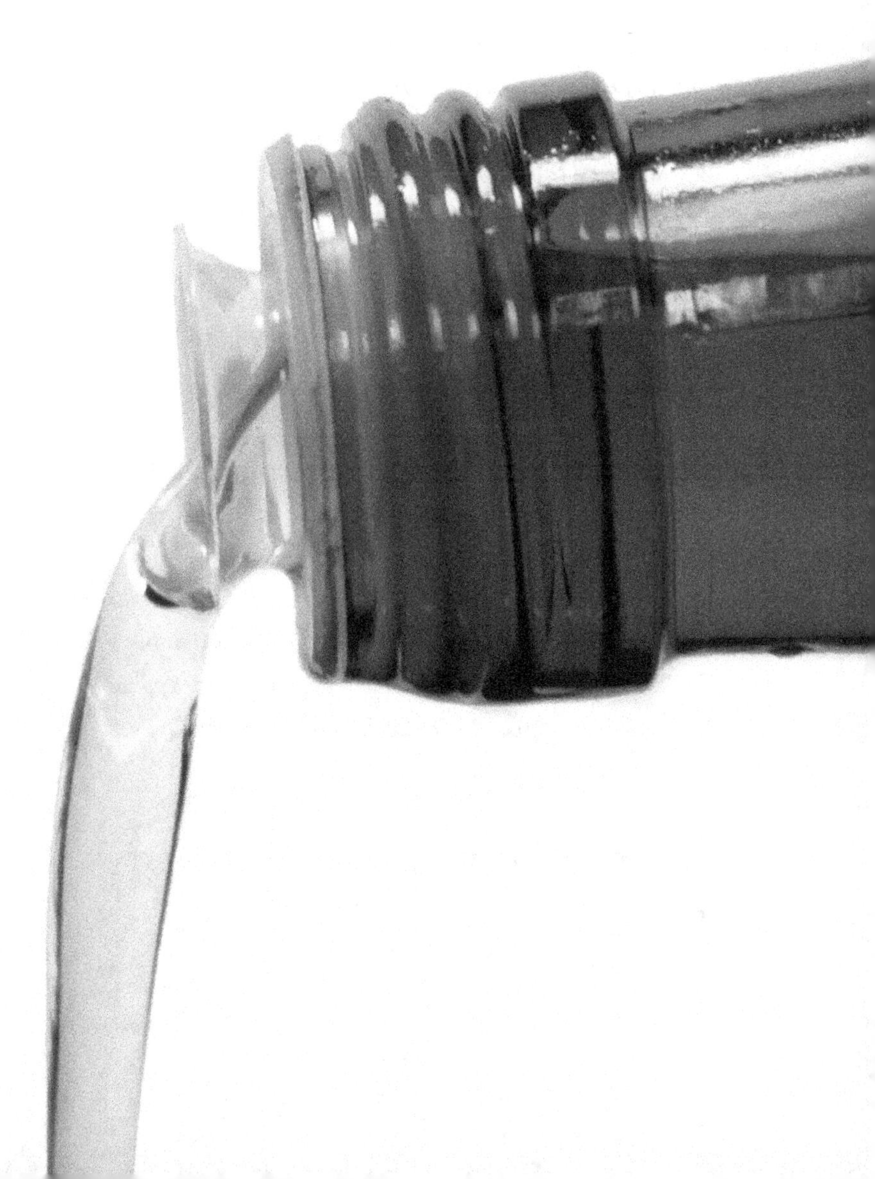

accept what is natural for them. It is important for kaphas to still try to maintain a normal body weight without starving themselves.

Obesity in kapha is mainly seen on the abdomen and thighs causing various problems with posture. Increased kapha also causes mucus formation around the breasts and lungs, which then spreads to different parts of the body and causes blockages in the ducts. These blockages contribute to increased fat accumulation around joints and tissues.

Kapha people are rarely physically active, although needing it to stimulate their metabolism and increase circulation. As kaphas are easily affected by high cholesterol and heart disease, they should exercise with caution and be mindful not to overwork while still challenging themselves.

As heat triggers the flow in kaphas, exercises that increase heat and make the body sweat are good. Kaphas need to be pushed to do exercises that are difficult and that they do not think they can do.

Sitting asanas increase kapha. Pranayamas that increase heat are beneficial before meditation.

*Vinyasas such as the sun salutation are good to start
the flow. Backward bending positions are also good as
they open up the chest, which is the area for kapha.
Backbends also increase circulation in the head, which
counteracts inertia. Forward bending positions should
generally be avoided by kaphas unless they are in need
of calming the nervous system.*

*Kaphas often suffer from slow digestion. Exercises, like
the arch, that initiate the flow at the navel region are
therefore particularly good. The plow is one of the best
positions to open up the lungs. Pranayamas initiate the
flow in both body and mind.*

*After asanas, kaphas should feel light and warm and
have increased circulation in the body. Chest and lungs
should be open and the mind should feel clear and alert.*

Seated poses:
*Simhasana(the lion) and in combination with pranay-
amas.*

The sun salutation:
At a fast pace.

Standing poses:
Virabhadrasana(warrior), Utthita hasta padangust-

*hasana(hand to toe stand), bakasana(crow), ardha
chandrasana(crescent position).*

Inverted poses:
*Adho mukha vrksasana(downward facing dog) sirsasa-
na(head stand), sarvangasana(shoulder stand).*

Backbends:
Ustrasana(camel pose), shalabasana(grasshopper pose).

Other:
*Shava udarakarshanasana(spinal rotation), ardha mat-
syendrasana(half spinal rotation), parvatasana(moun-
tain pose), halasana(plow pose).*

Shavasana:
Short.

PRANAYAMAS

*Yoga teaches us how to master prana and thus gain ac-
cess to its deeper powers. When we learn that, we are no
longer in need of external pleasure. In this way we take
control of our mind and can heal it and our body. A
knowledgeable Ayurveda doctor knows how to redirect
the prana in the body in order to heal the patient. In the
same way that food, herbs and other healing ways are
used to influence the prana.*

Pranayamas is one of the most central exercises in yoga and is the fourth step in classical yoga. The prana cleanses and revitalizes the body before meditation. With breathing exercises, you slow down and prolong your breath. This causes the life energy – the prana, to manifest itself.

Breathing exercises have a good effect on diseases that affect the respiratory organs, circulation and nervous system as well as fatigue and weak immune system. The whole body is affected by the exercises by massaging the internal organs. The circulation increases in the internal organs and is detoxified. Pranayamas also have a good effect on depression, stress and tension.

PRANA AND APANA

The apana associated with gravity moves downwards and results in disease, aging, death and unconsciousness. Prana associated with the elements of air and space moves upwards through our senses. By bringing these two energies together, we can strengthen our energy and awaken our higher abilities. Yogic exercises involve redirecting the apana upwards so that it meets the prana and pulling the prana down so that it meets the apana. This takes place at the solar plexus which is the seat of the prana.

Prana – inhalation.

Samana – hold your breath/contract.

Vyana – hold your breath/expand.

Udana – exhale/queeze out.

Apana – exhale/elimination.

PRANAYAMA AND PRANA AGNI

Pranayamas develop the fire of prana which is responsible for the body's combustion. This is done by holding your breath. Oxygen acts as food for pranaagni. The carbon dioxide that accompanies the exhalation is its residual product. Holding the breath cleanses our subtle body in the same way that fasting cleanses our physical. Prana agni gives power to Kundalini so it can continue its journey upwards and take with it prana and apana.

PRANAYAMAS AND DOSHAS

Pranayamas affect all doshas. Done correctly, they help balance vata, reduce kapha and counter pitta. Inhalation relates to kapha and has a constructive effect. Holding the breath in relates to the pitta and has a transforming effect. Exhalation relates to vata and has a reducing effect.

Breathing through the right nostril gives power to the pingala nadi and increases pitta. Breathing through the left nostril gives power to ida nadi and increases kapha.

A balanced breathing through both nostrils balances vata.

Kapha increases when you breathe through your mouth, which is generally advised against. However, there are some specific breathing exercises where you apply breathing through the mouth which can help the prana to be retained in the sushumna nadi.

VATA

Breathing through the right nostril is revitalizing for vata. Practice with intent in the morning for about ten to fifteen minutes. Breathing through the left nostril has a calming effect and calms the mind. Practice with intent in the evening to improve night sleep. Bhastrika can help with energizing and clarifying the mind but should be done carefully. End the exercise if dizziness occurs.

PITTA

Cooling pranayamas are best suited for pittas. Breathing through the left nostril is beneficial in the evening and in cases of feeling overheated or irritated. Shitali and sitkari pranayamas have a good effect on strong overheating, irritation and emotions.

KAPHA

Breathing through the right nostril is well suited for the

*morning as it reduces kapha. Bhastrika and kapalbhati
are excellent for kaphas especially for countering the
effects of colds(not fever), listlessness and depression.*

MEDITATION

*Meditation consists mostly of dharana (concentration),
dhyana(meditation) and samadhi(ecstasy). These three
steps belong to the inner aspect of the eight steps of
yoga. In Ayurveda, meditation is used for therapeutic
purposes, mainly to heal the mind and psychological
diseases but its effect also affects our physical body as
our physical body is also affected by our mental state. To
be able to meditate, the body, the prana and senses must
be in balance.*

*Both the body and the mind are made up of the five
elements. The body is composed of elements heavy in
character such as earth and water(kapha), which shapes
our body. The body's functions consist of the slightly
lighter elements and doshas. Pitta(fire) is responsible
for transformations within the body, while vata(air) is
responsible for the impulses between our brain and nerve impulses. The mind is made up of the lighter form of
vata(air and ether), which makes it volatile. The mind's
functions consist of the heavier elements: fire, water and
earth(pitta and kapha). Fire provides the mind with
perceptions, the water adds emotions and the earth*

connects the mind with the body. The mind is fast and in perpetual change.

Vatas are more quick-witted than other dosha types. It is easier for them to make new acquaintances(air) and be open to new experiences(ether). Vatas have very active senses and are always on the move somewhere. They are more often affected by mental and psychological imbalances.

Pitta is seen as the insightful part of the mind with the third eye of the mind relating to the element of fire. The fire of the mind is what is called buddhi(intellect and insight). Pitta types are often very intelligent with a good ability to focus and have sharp and clear thinking.

Kaphas feel emotions, love and devotion which are linked to our senses and the external character of the mind(manas). Bliss as the core of the mind is the highest form of kapha.

Meditation allows us to come in contact with our higher self and consciousness(atman and purusha). With the help of meditation, we can cleanse our subconscious from things that cause us suffering. Regardless of the meditation technique used, the purpose is to create the original stillness of our consciousness which is our true nature.

Meditation can help with:

– Psychological diseases.
– Difficulty falling asleep.
– Emotional disorders.
– Chronic diseases such as allergies and asthma that are affected by stress and hypersensitivity in the nervous system.
– Heart disease. According to ancient Vedic texts, our consciousness belongs to the heart. Calming the mind and strengthening the heart therefore go hand in hand.
– Pain relief by e.g. focusing on a mantra.
– Preparing for death and leaving the body.

MEDITATION FOR VATA

Meditation can help vatas with their hypersensitive and active mind to: provide better sleep, improve metabolism and strengthen the immune system. Caution must be exercised as meditation performed incorrectly can have the opposite effect on vatas and cause feelings of volatility. Vatas should first and foremost exercise their ability to concentrate. Techniques that include mantras and visualization are good because they saturate the mind instead of "emptying" it. Vatas should not try to calm the natural flow of thoughts but instead observe it and let it flow.

Preparation:
– Relaxing asanas help vata types sit for longer periods of time.
– Deep breathing exercises increase concentration by providing the body with prana.

Visualizations:
– Earth, fire and water.
– Mountains, lakes, flowers, fire and sunset.

Balancing colors:
– Gold and saffron help vata types achieve mental clarity.

Mantras:
– Ram, Shrim and Hrim.
During meditation or when vata seems to be out of balance.

Deities to meditate on:
– Durga and Tara give a feeling of security.
– Shiva and Vishnu give a feeling of security.
– Ganesha creates a sense of grounding.

Considering vata's anxious and fearful nature, devotion to a god or devotion for any teacher or guru is suitable. In this way, vatas can leave their worries and problems to someone else and get help and experience security at the same time.

Vatas need to learn to experience the contact with the eternal within itself, create stability and not worry about the changing world. Vatas need space, and peace and quiet to get away from the pace of their surroundings. Meditation on the true eternal helps to slow down one's thoughts.

MEDITATION FOR PITTA

Pitta people need meditation to release emotions such as aggression and anger. They often have a good ability to concentrate and it is easy for them to meditate. Mantra meditation is a great way for pittas to take advantage of their strong mental energy by focusing it on a goal. Pitta types must work to expand their mind and heart with the help of the inner light and thus gain insight into the truth. The meditation should provide stillness in the mind and heart of the pitta.

Preparation:
– Soothing asanas that do not create too much heat in the body.
– Shitali pranayama or breathing through the left nostril to cool the system.

Visualizations:
– Mountains, forests, lakes and seas.
– Rain clouds, flowers in cold colors, the moon and the stars.

Balancing colors:
– White, dark blue and green.

Affirmations:
– Devotion, love and forgiveness to balance the fire.
– Prayers for peace and love for other people.

Mantras:
– Shrim, Sham and Om. Recited silently.

Deities to meditate on:
– Lakshmi, Uma parvati, Shiva and Vishnu.

Pittas can be very critical and judgmental. They can use and transform this power by redirecting it to explore their inner self and expand their consciousness. Meditating on infinite space beyond all limitations is beneficial to their critical minds.

MEDITATION FOR KAPHA

Kaphas need meditation to free themselves from old emotional and mental patterns, and to counteract iner-

tia. Kaphas need a lot of encouragement and motivation to meditate so group meditation is usually best suited for them.

It is easy for kaphas to fall asleep and daydream so choosing an active form of meditation can help prevent this from happening. A combined form of meditation and activity with mantras or pranayamas is good.

Preparation:
– Powerful asanas that start the circulation in the body.
– Bhastrika pranayama or breathing through the right nostril.

Visualization:
– Fire, air and ether.
– Sun, wind, sky.

Balancing colors:
– Gold, blue and orange.

Affirmations:
– Which strengthens the connection to the higher self. Like for example. "In my true self I am independent and free, in nature and in space."

Mantras:
– Om, Hum and Aim.

Cleansing and stimulating, to be recited out loud.

Deities to meditate on:
– Shiva and Kali.Divinities of an angry nature that release emotions and reduce the ego.

Meditating on emptiness and the inner light creates more space and fire in the mind, which is beneficial for kaphas.

PULSE DIAGNOSTICS

In Ayurveda, various techniques are used to establish a diagnosis of one's health. These include analysis of heart rate, urine, feces, eyes, tongue, speech, skin, shape, and most importantly, the pulse. Taking one's pulse as a diagnostic tool has been used in Ayurveda since time immemorial. A well-experienced Ayurvedic physicist can use the pulse to assess prakruti(one's general constitution), vikruti(current imbalances in the doshas), subtle imbalances and other diseases.

You can read the pulse in different places in the body – e.g. in the armpit, ankle and wrist, of which the latter is the most common. This is done by placing the index finger, middle finger and ring finger on the upper side of the wrist(towards the thumb). The three fingers represent the three different doshas vata, pitta and kapha.

The index finger represents the vata dosha, the middle finger the pitta dosha, and the ring finger the kapha dosha. Each dosha has a characteristic pulse: from where the pulse starts, where on the finger it beats the strongest, from which direction it beats, and what quality the pulse has. Rishis use animal movement patterns to describe heart rate levels:

The vata pulse's movement pattern can be compared to how a cobra moves. It is fast, weak, cold, thin and disappears with pressure and is best felt under the index finger.

The pitta pulse's movement pattern can be compared to a frog. It is prominent, strong, warm, powerful, lifts the palpating finger and is best felt under the middle finger.

The kapha pulse's movement can be likened to a swimming swan. It is deep, slow, wide, wavy, dense, cold or hot, regular, and can be best felt under the ring finger.

THE SEVEN LEVELS OF THE PULSE

In Ayurveda, the pulse is divided into seven different levels, each of which tells us how we feel mentally, physically and spiritually. You can read the different levels by placing three palpating fingers on the wrist and changing pressure. The pulses provide the practitioner

*with vikruti(imbalances) that are present in our doshas
at the moment. Manas vikruti(manas: mind).*

Subdoshas.
*Each dosha(vata, pitta and kapha) has five subdoshas.
Each subdosha represents a particular aspect of our
physiology. In each subdosha, one of the five elements is
prominent.*

*Vata subdoshas: prana, udana, samana, vyana and
apana.*

*Pitta subdoshas: pachaka, ranjaka, alochaka, sadhaka
and bharajaka.*

*Kapha subdoshas: kledaka, avalambaka, bodhaka,
tarpaka and shleshaka.*

Prana, tejas and ojas.
*Prana is the essence of vata, tejas is the essence of pitta
and ojas is the essence of kapha.*

*Ojas are created during nutrition and are the main es-
sence of all tissues. Tejas can be compared to hormones
and amino acids. Prana, which is the vital life energy, is
responsible for the cooperation between cells.*

Dhatus represents our biological tissues such as plasma, blood tissues, muscle tissues, adipose tissues, bones, nerve tissues, male and female reproductive tissues.

Prakruti represents our basic psychosomatic and bio-logical constitution. Manas Prakruti(manas: sun). If a person says that they are, for example, a pitta person, they are not talking about any imbalance but about their basic constitution.

CHINESE MEDICINE

Pulse diagnostics is also an important part of Chinese medicine. However, Ayurvedic pulse diagnostics and Chinese differ somewhat. In Chinese technology, one can read forty-seven different aspects of the pulse, compared with the seven levels present in Ayurveda.

AYURVEDIC TREATMENTS

In Ayurvedic treatment, there are eight main disciplines, so-called ashtangas:

Internal medicine(kaya-chikitsa).
Pediatrics(kaumarabhrityam).
Surgery(shalya-chikitsa).
Eyes(shalakya-tantra).
The science of demonic obsession(bhuta-vidya). Has been called psychiatry.

Toxicology(agada-tantram).

Disease prevention, immunity enhancement and rejuve-
nation(rasayana).

Aphrodisiacs and improving the health of the
offspring(vajikaranam).

AYURVEDIC MASSAGE

Ayurvedic massage is used to treat a variety of diseases,
and for preventive purposes.

There are at least forty different types of Ayurvedic
massage which, along with a variety of other diagnostic
tools, are used by Ayurvedic doctors to treat diseases
and ill health.

Ayurvedic massage relieves pain, relaxes stiff muscles,
reduces swelling caused by joint inflammation, improves
blood circulation, increases stress resistance, provides
better sleep, increases athletic performance and provides
emotional benefits. With Ayurvedic massage, deeply
rooted toxins are released in joints and tissues, and then
eliminated through natural processes.

ABHYANGHA - AYURVEDIC OIL MASSAGE

Abhyangha(oil massage) is a common Ayurvedic
massage. Abhyanga is a therapeutic massage of about
forty-five minutes and is used to treat a large number of
diseases.

Abhyanga is often given by two therapists working on either side of the client, who is lying on a wooden bed. Particular attention is paid to the feet because there are marma points(nerve nodes) on the soles of the feet that are closely related to certain internal organs. The sole of the right foot is massaged with clockwise movement and the left foot counterclockwise.

During treatment, the client rests in seven standard positions. Abhyanga begins with the client sitting in an upright position, after which she lies flat on her back, turns to the right side, lies on her back again, turns to the left side, lies on her back again and finally returns to a sitting position. Abhyanga is an essential part of pancha karma therapy.

SHIROABHYANGA – AYURVEDIC HEAD MASSAGE

Shiroabhyanga is a head massage with roots in Ayurveda. The purpose of shiroabhyanga is not only to ward off stress but also to stimulate the body to heal itself. Various oils are usually included as a natural part of the treatment, to soothe the soul and care for the skin and hair. Shiroabhyanga is a head massage which, in addition to Ayurvedic contexts, is common in hair salons in India.

NASYAM - AYURVEDIC NASAL TREATMENT

Nasyam is an Ayurvedic treatment in which medicinal oils are administered through the nose to clear the throat, nose and head of harmful substances.

This treatment is used to treat migraines, headaches, mental disorders, prematurely graying hair and speech difficulties. Nasyam is also said to strengthen the mind and intellect and is included in pancha karma treatment.

PANCHA KARMA

Perhaps the most famous form of Ayurvedic treatment is pancha karma. Pancha karma, or literally "five actions" in Sanskrit, is a cleansing treatment to increase the metabolic process with appropriate diet, natural herbs and minerals. Pancha karma is used both for deep-rooted chronic diseases and for seasonal imbalances of the three elemental energies(doshas) pitta, vata and kapha. The purpose of the treatment is to make the body healthy by eliminating bodily waste products and achieving a balance between the doshas.

Pancha karma – five actions in three steps.
The five measures consist of: nasyan(nasal treatment), vamana(vomiting), virechana(detoxing), nirooha vasti (enemas with herbal decoctions), and sneha vasti(ene-

mas with herbal oils). After these treatments, hopefully the body has been cleansed of accumulated toxins.

Panchakarma is always performed in three stages: purva karma(pre-treatment), pradhana karma(primary treatment) and paschat karma(post-treatment). The patient who chooses any of the five treatments above must always undergo all three stages for the treatment to have the intended effect.

Step 1. Pre-treatment(purva karma).
Snehana(oil therapy) is an important preparatory treatment. Snehana is said to loosen toxins that are stuck in different places in the body and is often given with adapted herbal mixtures to treat an individual disease, but can also be given in a pure form without additives. Snehana is given early in the morning for a maximum of seven days and is said to help the transfer of toxins to the gastrointestinal tract so that it can be easily removed afterwards. If snehana is not given before pancha karma, the intended effect on the treatment will not be obtained.

Oil massage(abhyangha) is another important treatment in pancha karma.
Svedana is a therapy that induces sweating and is administered to the whole body or parts of the body

depending on the disease. Steam with added medicinal herbs is usually used, but can also be achieved by having the patient sit under the sun, while thirsty, hungry, and having their body covered with thick sheets; or by staying in a closed dark room. Svedana is said to dilate ducts in the body and thus helps move toxins to the gastrointestinal tract.

Step 2. Primary treatment(pradhana karma).
The toxins and slag products that reach the gastrointestinal tract are believed to be eliminated during the primary treatment.

One of the five primary treatments, vamana karma, is used for kapha diseases such as bronchitis, colds, coughs, asthma, sinusitis, and excess mucus. One to three days before vamana karma, one is treated with oil both internally and externally. Externally through abhyanga(Ayurvedic massage) and internally with ghee(shredded butter) in the diet.

Step 3. Post-treatment (paschat karma).
The finishing treatment consists of adapted diets, appropriate physical effort and intake of herbs to promote long-term health.

AYURVEDA AND SESAME OIL

Sesame oil is an oil that is extracted from sesame seeds and is most often used in cooking as a seasoning, but in Ayurveda it is also used for massage and skin care. It has been used for thousands of years in India due to its healing effects.

In Ayurveda, regular massage with sesame oil is recommended to achieve many health benefits. Ayurveda practitioners believe that massage with sesame oil cleanses; balances the lymphatic system and the endocrine system; lubricates; and softens muscles, tissues and joints. They also believe that the oil makes the skin radiant and youthful. Sesame oil is the best oil to use due to its ability to penetrate the skin and because it is generally recommended for all body constitutions, whether you are a vata, kapha or pitta.

According to Ayurveda, sesame oil is excellent because it is naturally antibacterial against common skin pathogens, such as staphylococci and streptococci, and against common skin fungi, such as athlete's foot. It is also naturally antiviral and anti-inflammatory.

Additionally, sesame oil is considered to relieve or cure psoriasis, dry scalp, irritated skin, skin rashes in teens, regulate pore enlargement; and heal or protect wounds.

AYURVEDIC MASSAGE IN THE HOME

How to do Ayurvedic oil massage at home.

1. Before starting the massage, warm the oil to body temperature or higher. Start by massaging your head. Dip your fingertips into the oil and massage the oil into the scalp. During the entire massage, use as much of the entire palm of your hand as possible, not just the fingertips. Since the head is one of the most important body parts to massage, feel free to spend a little more time there than for the other parts.

2. Gently lubricate the face and outer ears. Massage with the entire palm where possible. Massage your face and neck gently. Do not massage as strongly here as on other body parts.

3. Then go on to the neck and upper spine. Massage with open hands and light movements.

4. It is good if you first apply the oil on all body parts and then start again from the top and massage. In this way, the oil has time to stay on the skin for a longer time.

5. Continue with your arms. Massage with reciprocating movements(long up and down movements) along the long muscles and with circulating movements over the joints.

6. Proceed to the chest and abdomen. Massage over the heart with light circular motions. Massage the abdomen clockwise from the lower right side, upwards, to the lower left side.

7. Massage all parts of the back and spine as far as you can.

8. Continue with the legs. Massage with reciprocating movements along the large muscles and with circulating movements over the joints.

9. Finally, massage your feet. Just like the head, the feet are considered one of the most important body parts to massage. Feel free to spend a little more time here. Massage the soles of the feet with the entire palm.

10. Finish with a hot bath or shower.

www.ingramcontent.com/pod-product-compliance
Lightning Source LLC
LaVergne TN
LVHW041237200726
843507LV00013B/2723